## TABLE OF CONTENTS

**Anti Aging Techniques EXPOSED Vol 2**
Aging Beauty Secrets Revealed
©Copyright 2013 by Dr. Noah Pranksky

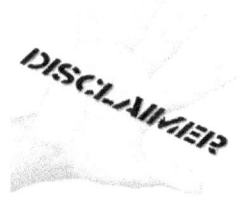

## DISCLAIMER AND TERMS OF USE AGREEMENT:

**(Please Read This Before Using This Book)**

ideas contained in this book, you are taking full responsibility for your actions.

The authors and publisher disclaim any warranties (express or implied), merchantability, or fitness for any particular purpose. The author and publisher shall in no event be held liable to any party for any direct, indirect, punitive, special, incidental or other consequential damages arising directly or indirectly from any use of this material, which is provided "as is", and without warranties. As always, the advice of a competent legal, tax, accounting, medical or other professional should be sought where applicable.

The authors and publisher do not warrant the performance, effectiveness or applicability of any sites listed or linked to in this book. All links are for information purposes only and are not warranted for content, accuracy or any other implied or explicit purpose. No part of this may be copied, or changed in any format, or used in any way other than what is outlined within this course under any circumstances. Violators will be prosecuted.

This book is © Copyrighted by ePubWealth.com.

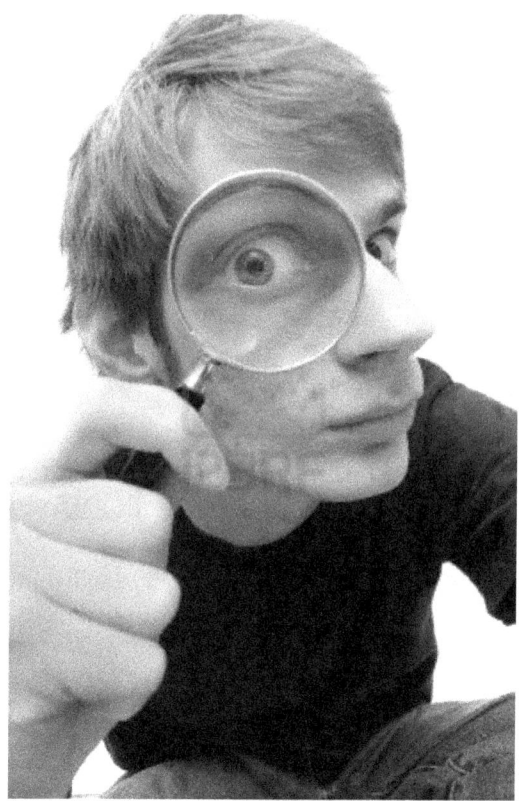

The mysteries of looking young are a much sought after topic. How do we retain or recapture our youth?

The facts are – once you reach the age of 40 – your body has forgotten what it feels like to be young. So, from a medical point of view, let's discuss the aging process.

The human body is made up of eighteen (18) chemical elements all of which are the identical elements found in soil. When we die, the same bio-flora and bacteria that sustained life are the very same elements that deteriorate the body in death causing it to return to its base elements.

Science tells us that the human body grows and develops from birth until about the age 20-22.

Physiologically speaking, the cause of this growth and development is the secretion of Human Growth Hormone (HGH) by the anterior lobe of the pituitary gland located in the rear of the skull.

Beginning in your early twenties, this very important gland slows down its production of HGH and the body begins to age.

This aging process is the actual deterioration of the body and in actuality we physically begin to die.

By the age of 40, the pituitary gland has pretty much ceased the production of HGH. Gray hair starts to grow, you begin to feel the effects of aging more so than any time in the past.

*(Special note: It is very popular in today's nutritional circles to tout the retardation of the aging process by using synthetic HGH, as well as various HGH precursor formulations. Synthetic HGH is used to treat dwarfism and I DO NOT recommend casual use of this substance without the advice of a licensed medical practitioner. It is very dangerous stuff! On the other hand, HGH precursors are relatively safe and natural formulations using an amino acid precursor base. In essence, this type*

*of precursor stimulates the pituitary gland to secrete more HGH.  This technology, dates back to 1982, and was developed through diabetes research.*

So, in essence, aging begins in our early 20s and progressively gets worse based on our lifestyle, our diets, our habits and our environment.

Here is how Oswald Chambers described our lives based on habits and environment:

**"We are what we are in the dark; all the rest is reputation.  What God looks at is what we are in the dark-the imaginations of our minds; the thoughts of our heart; the habits of our bodies, these are the things that mark us in God's sight."**

There is the "inner you" and an "outer you," which is what the world sees.  The physical or outer you is what we are concerned with here but, the outer you relies very heavily on the inner you...

**Scientists do not appear to see the difference between the matter part of an organism and the life part, which animates it.  They seem to think that the organism itself is life.  People suffer a similar problem of understanding.**

Life IS NOT what comes out of the body (the animated part of our existence); life is what goes into the body so we must pay special consideration to what we eat and ingest as well as our habits and lifestyle.

The scientific community often refers to the body as a "finely-tuned machine". The body IS NOT a machine! A machine functions on the totality of the parts that make up the machine. When a part breaks, the machine no longer functions. The human body is constantly renewing itself; new cells replace dying or dead cells. A machine cannot renew itself!

The human body is truly a marvel to behold!

The skin is an ever-changing organ that contains many specialized cells and structures. The skin functions as a protective barrier that interfaces with a sometimes-hostile environment. It is also very involved in maintaining the proper temperature for the body to function well. It gathers sensory information from the environment, and plays an active role in the immune system protecting us from disease. Understanding how the skin can function in these many ways starts with understanding the structure of the 3 layers of skin - the epidermis, dermis, and subcutaneous tissue.

### Epidermis
The outer layer of skin is called the epidermis. The thickness of the epidermis varies in different types of skin. It is the thinnest on the eyelids at .05 mm and the thickest on the palms and soles at 1.5 mm.

The epidermis is made up of 5 layers. From bottom to top the layers are named:

- stratum basale
- stratum spinosum

- stratum granulosum
- stratum licidum
- stratum corneum

The bottom layer - the stratum basale - has cells that are shaped like columns. In this layer the cells divide and push already formed cells into higher layers. As the cells move into the higher layers, they flatten and eventually die and are replaced by the underlying cells that are moving up; hence a constant renewal of the skin.

The top layer of the epidermis, the stratum corneum, is made of dead, flat skin cells that shed about every 2 weeks.

**Specialized Epidermal Cells**
The epidermis contains three types of specialized cells:

- The melanocyte produces pigment (melanin)
- The Langerhans' cell is the frontline defense of the immune system in the skin
- The Merkel's cell's function is not clearly known

**Dermis**
The thickness of the dermis varies depending on the location of the skin. It is .3 mm on the eyelid and 3.0 mm on the back. The dermis is composed of three types of tissue that are present throughout - not in layers. The types of tissue are:

- collagen
- elastic tissue
- reticular fibers

**Layers of the Dermis**

- The dermis' two layers are the papillary and reticular layers.
- The upper, papillary layer contains a thin arrangement of collagen fibers.
- The lower, reticular layer is thicker and made of thick collagen fibers that are arranged parallel to the surface of the skin.

**Specialized Dermal Cells**

- There are many specialized cells and structures in the dermis.
- The hair follicles reside here as are the erector pili muscle that attaches to each follicle.
- The follicle has two associated glands - Sebaceous (oil) glands and apocrine (scent) glands.
- This layer also contains eccrine (sweat) glands, but they are not associated with hair follicles.
- Blood vessels and nerves course through this layer. The nerves transmit sensations of pain, itch, and temperature.
- There are also specialized nerve cells called Meissner's and Vater-Pacini corpuscles that transmit the sensations of touch and pressure.

**Subcutaneous Tissue**
The subcutaneous layer is made up mostly of fat and connective tissue that houses larger blood vessels and nerves. This layer is important is the regulation of

temperature of the skin itself and the body. The size of this layer varies throughout the body and from person to person.

The complicated structure of the skin has many functions. If any of the structures in the skin are not working properly, a rash or abnormal sensation is the result. The whole specialty of dermatology is devoted to understanding the skin, what can go wrong, and what to do if something does go wrong.

## Chapter 1 - How Skin Ages

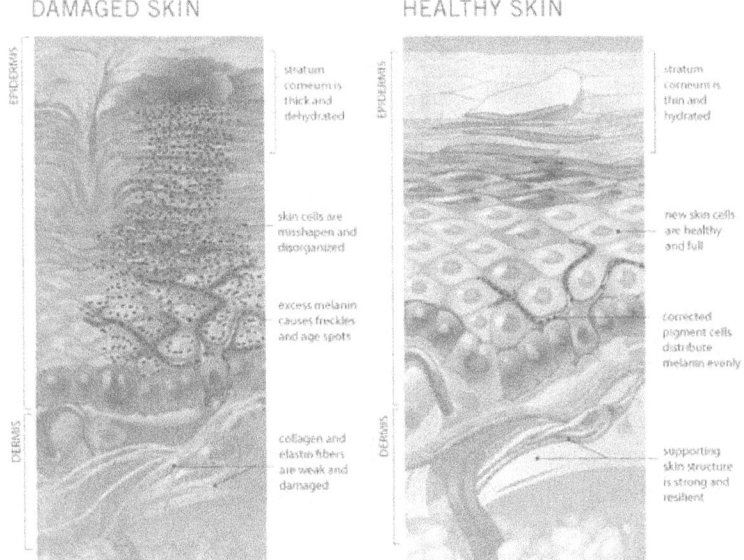

DAMAGED SKIN

EPIDERMIS

stratum corneum is thick and dehydrated

skin cells are misshapen and disorganized

excess melanin causes freckles and age spots

DERMIS

collagen and elastin fibers are weak and damaged

HEALTHY SKIN

EPIDERMIS

stratum corneum is thin and hydrated

new skin cells are healthy and full

corrected pigment cells distribute melanin evenly

DERMIS

supporting skin structure is strong and resilient

Our skin becomes less flexible and less elastic as we age. The skin is the largest organ in the human body! Like other bodily organs, aging makes them less flexible and elastic such as your heart muscle, your arteries, even your eyes, etc.

Wrinkles and other signs of aging, which are the physical effects of aging, occur with aging. The two main reasons for the physical effects of aging are the body's natural processes and its exposure to the environment. Understanding why skin ages can point to some simple anti-aging skin care techniques.

### Natural Aging:

As stated above, beginning in our 20s, the skin begins to slowly and steadily age. Dead skin cells are not replaced as quickly, collagen production slows and our skin loses elasticity. Signs of this type of aging include:

- fine wrinkles
- thinner skin
- a 'hollow' look due to loss of fat below the skin
- sagging skin, due to bone shrinkage and muscle atrophy
- dry, itchy skin

### Exposure-Related Aging:

Exposed skin can also suffer damage. The sun's UV rays cause the most damage. Other external sources of skin aging include repeated sleeping positions, facial expressions and smoking. Anti aging skin care should involve reducing exposure to sunlight and the use of face creams with UV protection.

### Sleeping Positions:

Sleep lines can occur when people sleep on their sides or stomachs. These often appear on the sides of the face or the forehead as a result of sleeping each night in contact with the pillow. People who sleep on their backs will not get sleep lines.

### Facial Expressions:

Grooves under the skin can be caused by repetitive facial movements that eventually become wrinkles. Laugh lines, worry lines and other wrinkles can be caused this way.

## Gravity:

Our appearance over time changes by the slow, steady pull on our body caused by gravity. Starting in our 50s, nose tips being to droop, ears become longer, eyelids fall, and jowls may form.

## Smoking:

Some of the most severe damage to the skin is caused by smoking and is also the cause of many of the outward signs of aging; even turn a smoker's skin yellow. If a smoker quits, some of these signs may be reduced or even vanish. Quitting smoking is the single best anti aging skin care technique anyone can do. Long-term cigarette smoking adds to the aging of the skin because of the chemical changes it causes. Further damage can be avoided by stopping smoking.

## Sunlight:

'Photoaging' is the term used by dermatologists to describe the effects of sunlight on unprotected skin. These effects include:

- skin cancer
- freckles
- age spots
- spider veins
- rough skin
- blotchiness

To protect your skin from premature aging and skin cancer:

- Cover: Try to cover your body to reduce your exposure to sunlight. Wear a hat, long pants and a long-sleeved shirt if you will be outdoors long.
- Sunscreen: Wear sunscreen when you are outdoors, even if it is cloudy or in the wintertime.
- No Tanning: Do not sunbathe or use tanning booths.

**Skin Problems of the Elderly**

The elderly have special consideration when it comes to caring for the skin and the older you get; the more important it is to take care of your skin. Your skin changes as you age and some of these changes are not necessarily changes over time. It becomes thinner and begins to sag, causing wrinkles. It injures more easily and heals more slowly. The skin also loses its ability to moisturize itself.

Aging adults suffer more from dry, itchy skin is and is an annoying but common problem in aging adults. To avoid dry skin, try the following:

- take only 2 to 3 short baths or showers a week; use warm water (not hot)
- always shower or bathe immediately after getting out of a pool or spa that has chlorine in it
- use soaps made for dry skin, such as glycerin soap with cleansing cream
- rinse well after using soaps

- Apply lotion immediately after drying skin, while it is still slightly moist; this helps lock in moisture (Be sure the skin is not too wet or you can get a fungal infection.)
- apply lotion all over your body at bedtime; put gloves and socks on after applying lotion to retain moisture
- drink more liquids
- use a humidifier during the winter and in dry climates
- avoid alcohol, spicy food, and caffeine
- avoid dry places, such as saunas and the desert

**Stasis Dermatitis** is a skin condition that results in redness, swelling, tenderness, and dry scaly skin. It is found more often in women over the age of 50. The condition is the result of water pooling in the lower leg due to poor blood flow in the veins. Scratching the dry skin causes bruises, ulcers, and more damage to the leg. Treatments include raising the leg, wrapping the leg with an elastic bandage (be sure it is not tight enough to cut off the circulation), and medication.

**Exfoliative dermatitis** is excessive peeling or shedding of the skin. It is more common in men over the age of 40. The skin may feel tight or hair may be lost in that area. It may be caused by drug reactions, leukemia, malignancies, and other immune deficiencies. Treatments include bed rest, lukewarm soaks or baths, creams and lotions, prescription medications (such as antihistamines or steroids), and rubbing the skin gently when it itches, instead of scratching. Scratching may open the skin and lead to infection.

Sun damage can cause problems in skin appearance, such as roughness, wrinkles, "age" or "liver" spots, and dilated blood vessels, and skin cancers. Even if you already have sun damage, you are never too old to prevent further damage. Be sure to avoid being in the sun between 10 AM and 4 PM. Wear a hat with a wide brim and dark colored, tightly woven clothes that cover your arms and legs. Avoid tanning salons and sun lamps.

The use of a sunscreen is mandatory if you are going to be in the sun for more than 20 minutes. One ounce, enough to fill a shot glass, is the amount needed to completely cover the body. Be sure it has a Sun Protection Factor (SPF) of 15 or higher with UVA and UVB protection. Apply sunscreen well to the face, ears, hands and arms 15 to 20 minutes before going outdoors. Re-apply every 2 hours or immediately after swimming or strenuous activity.

There are a few cancers that are more common in aging skin. Some are caused by years of excessive sun exposure. Others may be because cancer runs in your family or you inherited a type of skin that increases the risk of skin cancer.

It is important to examine your skin routinely for new spots or changes because skin cancer is the most common form of cancer in the United States. Look for:

- a single, flat or slightly indented, hard lesion; it may be yellow or white with irregular edges
- a red, scaly area that slowly enlarges

- a change in the color, shape or size of a mole; or if a mole begins to bleed
- an open area that does not heal and
- any new skin growth

Melanoma is the most serious type of skin cancer and it usually starts in a mole. Most melanomas can be identified using the following A-B-C-D criteria.

**A** = Asymmetry (the left side of the lesion is not the same as the right side)

**B** = Border Irregularity (the edges are irregular, ragged, or poorly defined)

**C** = Color (the color is not the same all over; there may be patches of tan, brown, black, pink, white or blue)

**D** = Diameter (the area is larger than a pencil eraser or is growing)

You cannot detect skin cancer yourself. Be sure to have any suspicious skin area examined by a healthcare provider. Also be sure to talk with your provider if a skin problem does not get better with home care.

## Chapter 2 - Perfect Skin Dos and Don'ts

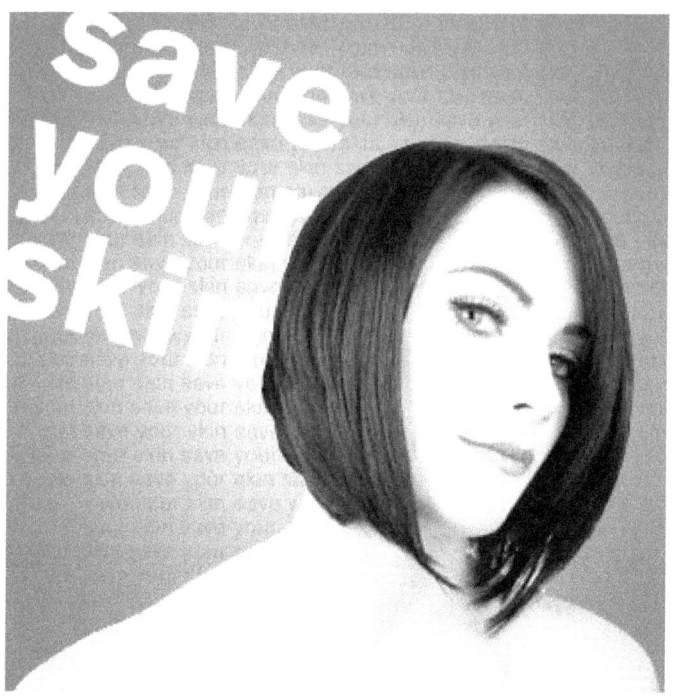

If youth only knew; if age only could...young people believe in their 20s or early 30s that they can't possibly have aging skin yet. Wrong! Your skin's "youthfulness" has less to do with age than how it's been treated, so if exposed to sun, smoke and stress, your skin will start "acting old," losing collagen, glow and elasticity. Lines will develop prematurely and your skin may look dull and "blah."

It's easier to prevent damage than to repair it, but the good news is you can put the brakes on prematurely aging skin and you can reverse the aging process, well, to a point.

### 5 Dos and 5 Don'ts to Help Slow the Aging Skin Process

**Do stop smoking.** Ever notice the skin of a lifelong smoker? It can appear wrinkly like a squashed paper bag. Nicotine constricts blood vessels and decreases the flow of oxygen to the skin.

**Do use a retinoid every day or every few days.** A daily application of a prescription retinoid lotion such as Retin-A or Tazorac can give you a more youthful look. Dermatologists claim that retinoid is the one anti-aging product that really works.

If you suffer from dull skin; your complexion has a white cast, a dull pallor then try Retin-A. After using the product for a few weeks and going through the period where the skin turns red and peels, you will see amazing results.

AHAs, when used properly, not only rid your face of dead skin, but can take 10 years off as well by reducing fine lines.

(Keep in mind these products do NOT shrink pores. Your pore size is completely hereditary, so don't believe promises of permanent reduction).

Over-the-counter options such as RoC Deep Wrinkle Night Cream are good, but prescription creams work the best.

Extra tip: You must stay out of the sun if you use retinoids. You are extra-susceptible to sunburns.

**Do give yourself a facial once a week.** Practice At-Home Facials; your skin will never look better. Facials take only about 30-minutes and include cleansing, exfoliation via a facial scrub, a hydrating mask, a quick steam and moisturizer.

**Do wear sunscreen every day, rain or shine.** You've had it ingrained in your head since youth, but seriously, even in winter it can take just 20 minutes of unprotected sun exposure to damage the skin.

By the way, one of the many MYTHs is that we receive 80 percent of our lifetime sun damage occurs before age 18, according to O Magazine. Katie Rodan, MD, adjunct professor of dermatology at Stanford University School of Medicine, says in O that this myth stands officially debunked and studies indicate we get only 23 percent of total UV exposure by age 18.

**Do shield your windows.** The average commuter gets 200 hours of sun exposure each year and 80 percent of sun exposure is through car windows, according to Boston dermatologist Ranella Hirsch in Harper's Bazaar. To protect your skin against sun damage (the leading cause of aging skin), invest in a window shield like Solar

Gard. Shields with SPF 285 can block UVA and UVB rays by 99 percent.

**You saw the 5 "dos" for perfect skin care. Now here are 5 don'ts:**

**Don't pull and rub your skin.** Aging skin has been under attack by UV rays, stress and carbon monoxide so don't stress it more by pulling on it.

**Don't forget to moisturize.** While it's a myth that wrinkles are caused by dry skin, moisturizing can improve the appearance of lines by temporarily plumping them up. Also consider a good eye cream. Eye creams are controversial because some pros claim they don't really do anything, but many women swear by them.

*Extra tip: Moisturizers are best used on damp skin. They lock the moisture in. Dr. Dennis Gross doesn't use tap water when washing skin because of harsh minerals found in many city water sources. Instead, he rinses off with Evian water.*

**Don't ignore your neck and chest.** The neck and chest are first to show the signs of aging (they have fewer oil glands), yet most of us ignore them. Look for moisturizers that have age-fighting ingredients like vitamin A (retinols), kinetin, copper or vitamin C.

**Don't tan.** Even if wrinkles haven't shown up yet, you need to stop tanning now because they will. Once the signs of aging appear, you'll be spending a lot of money to reverse it. So if you do have sun damage?

Many spas and dermatologists provide pricey fixes with photo rejuvenation such as pulsed light treatments that can reverse the damage. If you do have brown spots, treat them with lemon juice diluted with water, according to NY dermatologist Jessica Krant in Harper's Bazaar. Krant suggests applying the mixture with a Q-tip nightly, gradually increasing it twice daily until sun spots fade away.

**Don't sporadically take care of your skin.** Be sure to cleanse your face every night to avoid clogged pores and to wash away all the pollution your skin has been subjected to and received.

Also keep up your anti-aging regimens for the best effects. You may suffer redness and a bit of peeling at first, but this is normal. To get the full effects of acid peels, retinoids, AHAs, and moisturizers you have to keep at it. The initial benefits will go away if you stop using them.

## Chapter 3 - Anti Aging Skin Care – Prevent and Treat Wrinkles

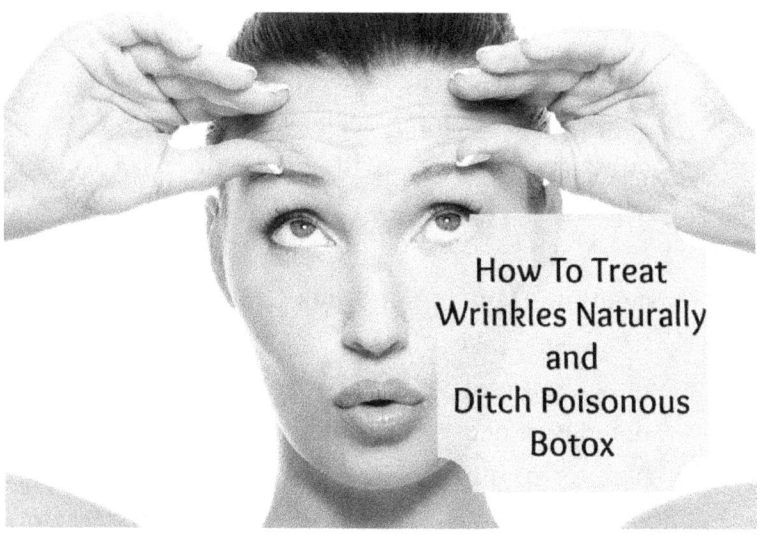

The number one target of anti aging skin care products is WRINKLES. Before discussing what works and what doesn't work with wrinkles, it is important to understand how wrinkles happen and what anti aging means.

### The Main Cause of Wrinkles – Sunlight

The real cause of wrinkles isn't aging but mostly by sunlight. UV rays from the sun penetrate your skin and damage fibers in your skin called elastin. As the elastin weakens, your skin becomes less elastic and losing its ability to snap back after being stretched. This results in wrinkles, especially in parts of your skin that get stretched and move a lot like around your eyes, mouth and nose.

**Gravity – It Sucks (LOL)**
Gravity makes you look older; as the elastin weakens through sun damage and as other changes in your skin happen due to aging such as less fat and less supportive structure. Gravity will pull your skin down causing sagging.

**Smoking Makes You Look Older**
Smoking makes you look older, lots older and is the direct cause of wrinkles in your skin through damage to the elastin and by depriving skin cells of oxygen. When pictures of smokers and non-smokers who are the same age are put next to each other, the smokers are always thought to be older. The more cigarettes smoked, the older the appearance.

**Anti Aging and Anti Wrinkle Skin Care Products**
Lots of products are available that claim to reduce and prevent wrinkles. Most of them don't work and most of the claims haven't been scientifically proven. Typically, the label will have some complex pseudo-scientific jargon about antioxidants, nutrients and other things that supposedly make your skin look younger. These claims are almost entirely untrue although some preliminary

research shows potential in special formulations that are not yet available over the counter.

NOTE: According to the NIH (National Institutes of Health) and the American Academy of Dermatology, most over-the-counter anti aging skin care products that target wrinkles merely soothe dry skin. This means they feel very nice going on, but do not reduce those wrinkles at all.

### Tretinoin Cream – One of the Best Anti Aging Skin Care Product

Tretinoin cream (Renova) is created from vitamin A and available with a prescription to treat sun damage and wrinkles as well as age spots and roughness by stimulating the skin to produce collagen (a substance that gives the skin structure). This cream is usually prescribed for people who have sun damage even after taking normal precautions to limit their exposure to UV rays. There are over-the-counter versions of various vitamin A-based anti aging skin care products. These have not been evaluated extensively and certainly do not work as well as the prescription versions.

### Reversing Sun Damage and Erasing Wrinkles Using Laser Technology

Two other treatment protocols have also been approved to treat sun damage and wrinkles - Carbon dioxide and erbium lasers. Use of these lasers is considered minor surgery and is done under anesthesia. This is an expensive process and is used in extreme cases.

### For Wrinkle and Sun Damage Removal Use Alpha Hydroxy Acids

Alpha hydroxyl acids may help eliminate the signs of aging such as wrinkles, age spots and sun damage. The use of alpha hydroxyl acids causes the user to become more sensitive to UV light and risk even more sun damage. Users should minimize their exposure to sunlight through using sunscreen and avoiding the sun. The long-term effects of this treatment are unknown.

### The Bottom Line is To Protect Against The Sun

The best anti aging skin care product available and reasonably inexpensive is still sunscreen. These other techniques and products mentioned herein are for extreme cases. If you are interested in them, talk to a qualified dermatologist but still be cautious. These treatments are expensive and not often covered by insurance.

### Facts on Anti Aging Skin Care and Anti Aging Skin Care Products

There are many anti aging skin care products and the marketplace is flooded with them making it very difficult to evaluate. Anti aging skin care products sell very well as aging is a primary concern for most people. We all want to look younger and hide the effects of aging on our skin.

But which of the techniques and methods really work?

How effective are anti aging skin care products?

Is it worth it to pay extra for products that claim to help reverse aging through antioxidants, mushrooms, enzymes and other scientifically sound approaches?

Let's examine some of the products and claims but care must always be exercise in evaluating and choosing any product and to be safe, consult your local dermatologist.

## Chapter 4 - The Facts on Anti Aging Skin Care Products

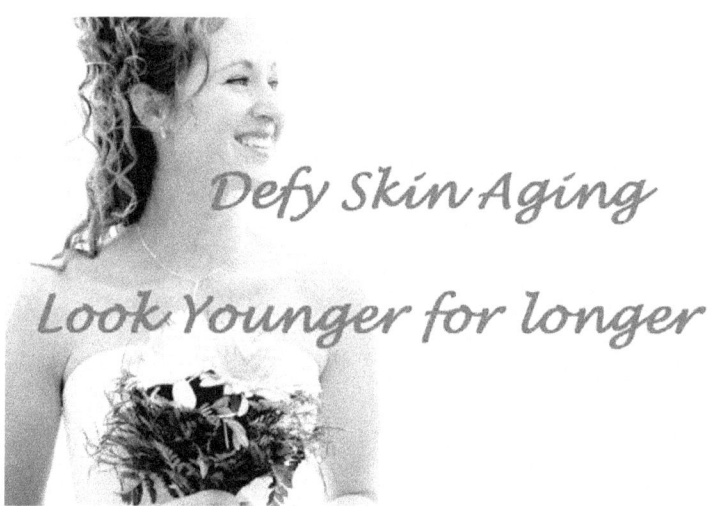

*Defy Skin Aging*

*Look Younger for longer*

Most information offered on anti aging skin care is involved in trying to sell you something so start your search for information at the National Institutes of Health's National Institute on Aging (the U.S.'s premier institution for the scientific study of aging).

You will find information on why skin ages and which products has been FDA approved for things like reversing wrinkles or treating age spots (these are usually prescription anti aging skin care products).

Here's what I found:

**Why Skin Ages - The Basics of Anti Aging Skin Care**

Exposure to UV light from the sun is the primary cause of aging skin. UV light batters our skin's cells with energy that can penetrate the cell walls and causes changes in cellular structure (and even in the DNA). Over time, this adds up to wrinkles, age spots, dry skin and more. Basically, exposure to sunlight over years and years makes the skin thinner and creates in skin appearance that we link to aging. Just think about it, most of the places where we are concerned about skin aging (face and hands) are the places that are most exposed to sunlight during our lives.

## Anti Aging Skin Care Problems (and What Really Works to Help Them)

As we age, we all face the same problems with our skin. There are thousands of products on the market that claim to help. In fact, most anti aging skin care problems really don't do anything to "make your skin younger," they just cover up the damage done. These anti aging skin care products are expensive but most are harmless (and do not work as they claim). Here's an overview of some of the common anti aging skin care problems and what to do about them:

**Wrinkles:** Wrinkles are a major target of anti aging skin care products. Wrinkles are caused by primarily two things: UV light from the sun and smoking. Both these things you can avoid. UV light exposure can be avoided (or greatly lessened) by avoiding spending lots of time in the sun and being sure to use sunscreen. Smoking can be avoiding by quitting smoking and making sure you are not exposed to second-hand smoke (for help quitting smoking, see our excellent site on smoking cessation).

**Dry Skin and Itching:** Dry skin and itching is a problem that many increases with age. Part of the reason that dry skin and itching are problems for older people is that, as you age, sweat and oil glands in your skin are lost. This results in dry skin and all the problems (like itching) linked with it. Creams, ointments and lotions can all help relieve dry and itching skin. You should also avoid using too much soap, taking too many baths and using too much perfume. All these things can dry the skin more. Anti aging skin care here mostly alleviates the symptoms, but does not "fix" the problem of dry skin.

**Age Spots:** These flat, brown spots are caused by exposure to the sun. They appear on areas of the body most exposed to sunlight like the face, arms and hands. The chances of getting age spots increase with age. Some anti aging skin care treatments exist to fade the age spots. Most important, sunscreen can help prevent further damage or increase in age spots.

**Bruising:** Another common skin problem linked to increased age is bruising easily. This is because the skin becomes thinner with age (again due to exposure to UV light and sun damage). In addition, some medications can cause the skin to bruise more easily.

**Skin Cancer:** Skin cancer is the most common form of cancer in the U.S. Almost 50% of Americans older than

65 develop skin cancer at least once in their life. To me, that number is rather shocking. It is critically important to routinely check your skin for skin cancer and have your skin checked by a dermatologist on a regular basis. Luckily, most skin cancer is easily treated, especially if caught early.

# Chapter 5 - Best Anti Aging Skin Care Methods

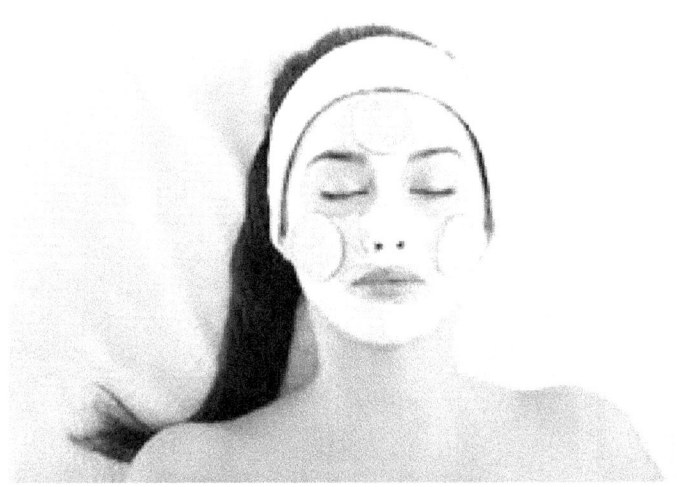

Anti aging skin care products should all have one thing in common: sunscreen. Sun damage is behind almost all of the signs of aging skin such as wrinkles and age spots. To prevent damage to your skin from aging, be sure that sunscreen is your number one anti aging skin care product. Choose a sunscreen with an SPF rating of at least 15 (use a sunscreen with a higher rating if you plan to be in the sun for a longer period of time). Also, be sure that you use a broad-spectrum sunscreen that protects your skin from damage from UVA and UVB rays. Finally, be sure that your sunscreen is water resistant even if you are not planning on swimming –- your sweat alone undoes the protection of non-water resistance sunscreens.

All the ointments, moisturizers and creams in the world can't compare to the anti aging effectiveness of ordinary sunscreen. Here are some other tips to keep looking young:

**Avoid the Sun:** Sunscreen is great, but if you can avoid long exposure to the sun that is even better. Don't spend a whole day at the beach in the beating sun. Limit your time out in the sun and your skin will age better.

**Wear Protective Clothing:** If you have to be in sun, do your best to keep the sun off your body. Wear long sleeved shirts and pants. A hat with a wide brim is great to protect your head and your face, neck and shoulders.

**Wear Sunglasses:** Your eyes can be damaged by UV light as well as your skin. Be sure to wear sunglasses that protect against 99% or more of UV rays.

**Avoid Artificial Tanning**: Sunlamps and tanning beds are just asking for trouble –- don't use them. They will damage your skin and speed your skins aging while increasing your risk for skin cancer. Artificial tanning lotions and make-up actually do provide some minimal protection from UV rays. But the effect is minimal and short-lasting. Your skin may look darker, but you have none of the protection of a real tan (and people often don't bother with sunscreen and tanning make-up together because it just ends up a creamy mess). Finally, avoid anything marketed as a tanning pill. These pills basically turn your skin orange and the long-term safety of high doses of tanning pills is unknown.

**Check Your Skin:** Almost of 50% of people who make it to age 65 will have skin cancer in their lifetime. You need to check your skin often for any signs of skin cancer as well as see a dermatologist regularly for a skin check. Learn how to do a skin self-check.

**Anti-aging Skin Care Tips**

Let's begin by breaking down our skin by decade; the following steps are something you should *always* do no matter your age or decade.

- Practice Sun safety
- Resurface
- Drink Water
- Eat well
- Pro-active stress relief

**20's** – Things begin to slow. For example, new skin cell production slows down by a rate of four times as cells go from a complete turnover every five to seven days to every 21 days.
This means that fine lines begin to develop around the eyes and mouth and photo damage starts showing in the form of freckles and spots.

**Tips for the 20's:**

- Some form of mild resurfacing needs to start. Do this at least two times per week.
- Daily sun protection (rain or shine)
- Begin to introduce antioxidants into regimen for extra protection. The antioxidants will also help

cells that are not fully damaged further protect themselves.

**The skin care routine established in your 20's is your staple. You'll want to continue that routine and add to it in your 30's and beyond.**

**30's** – This is the decade when stress becomes a factor on the skin. People are multi-tasking more; they are planning weddings, having babies, establishing themselves into careers, etc.
The cell turnover cycle has slowed to 28 days and pre-menopausal build-up starts to show on the skin.

When the pre-menopausal hormones are combined with stress, the effects on the skin include: adult onset acne, hormone-induced pigmentation, darkening of the skin above the lips, and fine lines becoming fuller.

**Tips for the 30's:**

- Practice pro-active stress reduction techniques such as Yoga, Pilates and meditation.
- Anti-inflammatory products (DHAs) should be added to regimen. These include mango, shea butter and salicylic acid.
- May want to start an actual treatment program for hyperpigmentation that combines daily resurfacing with professional treatments.

**Take what you did the 20's and 30's and add...**

**40's** – Welcome to the decade of defense! Cells now turn over every 45 days, so nourishing and protecting the skin is critical. The skin is drier and does not produce as many elastins.

**Tips for the 40's:**

- Daily resurfacing that includes regular in-clinic treatments (six times per year) and at home.
- Skin Growth Factors, Vitamin C, and Peptides should be added to boost collagen and elastin.

**When you hit the 50's, you are taking the skin care lessons that you've been doing since you were 20 and add...**

**50's** – It now takes two months (60 days) for cells to turn over. The skin is definitely not as lifted or tight.

**Tips for the 50s:**

- Non-invasive procedures may be considered including fillers that use natural substances to replenish what nature is no longer producing/
- Skin will be very dry. Hydration is key through moisturizers, lots of water and healthy food.

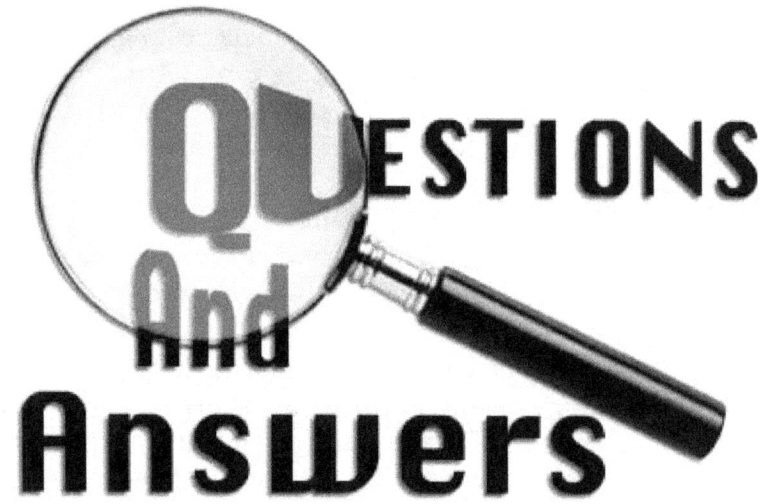

## 1. Do Hair Dyes Cause Cancer?

If your hair is going gray, you may be one of the estimated one-third of adult women – and one-tenth of adult men – who decide to cover it up with chemical color. The treatments range from an occasional set of reverse highlights that put darker color back into hair, all the way to coloring roots to eliminate gray every three weeks.

Some research data have suggested a higher incidence of certain cancers among hairdressers and barbers who use these preparations in their workplace, and among people who use them at home. Other studies have shown no link.

**Types of Hair Color**: There are a variety of products available to color aging hair. Temporary tints are easily washed out because they are not absorbed by the outer layer, or cuticle, of the hair shaft. Semi-permanent colors do penetrate and stain the cuticle, lasting up to six to 10 shampoos. Permanent dyes are by far the most popular, making up about 80% of the market. They last the longest by creating colored molecules within the hair shaft itself.

**Safety Concerns**: In the mid-1970s some research concluded that components of permanent hair dyes, including some aromatic amines, did cause cancer in animals. Consequently, most manufacturers removed those ingredients by 1980, so the U.S. Food and Drug Administration (FDA) and National Cancer Institute's summaries of health research on hair dyes often stipulate dangers associated with use prior to, or after, that year.

Unfortunately, there have been few studies since then that has firmly established a risk – or lack of risk – of cancer associated with hair dyes. In addition, the research that does exist doesn't always distinguish between the type of dye (temporary, semi-permanent, permanent) used by its subjects or the frequency of application. A person coloring roots every few weeks has a much greater chemical exposure than someone using a temporary rinse every few months. The main areas of research involve bladder cancer, marrow and blood cancers such as non-Hodgkin lymphoma and leukemia, and breast cancer.

Some studies have discovered a link between permanent dyes and bladder cancer, especially among long-term (more than 15 years) home users. By contrast, a large 2003 Swedish study of more than 45,000 male and female hairdressers found no increase in bladder cancers.

Other research on dyes and blood and bone marrow cancers, like non-Hodgkin lymphoma and leukemia, has also shown conflicting results. A 2007 review of four research projects, involving a total of more than 10,000 women, found that increases in one type of non-Hodgkin lymphoma were found only in women who began using hair dye before 1980, with the exception of an increase in follicular lymphoma among female users of dark-colored dye, who began coloring after 1980. Dark colors contain more of the aromatic amines, which make up the colorless "intermediate" component of the dye.

No link between hair dyes and breast cancer has been found.

**2. Birth defects**: Another question arises for many women regarding the risk of birth defects, either through personal use or exposure in the workplace. Some animal studies have shown teratogenic – or birth defect-causing – effects with very high doses. No birth defects have been linked in human use, however, probably because the absorption of chemicals through the skin is very limited.

Still, to err on the side of caution, doctors at the Motherisk Program at Toronto's Hospital for Sick Children recommend that women limit coloring their own hair to three to four times during a pregnancy. For hairdressers while pregnant, Motherisk advises wearing gloves and working in a well-ventilated area for no more than 35 hours per week.

Given some conflicting research results for hair dyes and cancer in general, the FDA issues the following guidelines for safe use:

- Leave hair dye on for only the recommended duration.
- Wear gloves when coloring hair.
- Rinse scalp well with water after coloring.
- Never mix different hair color products.
- Avoid other problems, such as contact dermatitis or hair dye allergies, by following all package instructions and warnings.

## 3. Does Aging Have to Make Me Look Old?

Aging doesn't have to make you look old. A lot of the changes to our skin and body due to aging are really an accumulation of damage from the ultraviolet light of the sun over years and years of exposure. You can prevent this damage and slow the aging of your skin through these simple steps:

**Use sunscreen** - The best idea here is a daily facial and hand cream that contains some level of UV protection. Get in the habit of putting it on every morning. But, if you are going to be out in the sun, use additional protection as well. Sunscreen is the single best anti aging skin care product you can use.

**Limit sun exposure** - As important as sunscreen is, you also want to make sure that you don't spend too much time in the sun. Pay special attention to your sun exposure as you go through the day doing routine things like walking your dog or gardening.

**Don't forget your hands** - Having sun damage on your hands can make you look older than you are. Don't forget to protect your hands from the damage of ultraviolet radiation.

**Do a skin check** - A skin cancer check won't make you look younger, but it can increase your life expectancy. Skin cancer is the most common cancer in the U.S. but the good news is that it is usually treatable if caught early. Follow these skin cancer screening guidelines.

### 4. Why Your Hair Goes Gray?

Gray hair has always been something of a mystery. Sure, as people age, they go gray – everybody knows that. But up until recently, no one really understood why gray hair is a common "side effect" of aging. There are all sorts of "beliefs" around the causes of gray hair like too much stress or teenagers.

### Researchers Take On Gray Hair

One of the reasons that we know so little about the causes of gray hair is because no one has really tried to figure it out. But now, with some many people aging and interested in looking younger, the business case for figuring out gray hair is very becoming compelling.

**Here is what they have figured out: Hydrogen Peroxide Causes Gray Hair**

As you age, the amount of hydrogen peroxide in your hair increases. This happens because hydrogen peroxide (believe it or not) is produced naturally in your body. When levels in hair build up, it (essentially) bleaches out your normal hair color and leaves with gray hair.

**Why Does Hydrogen Peroxide Build Up and Cause Gray Hair?**

What happens is that an enzyme in your body (called catalase) usually breaks down the hydrogen peroxide. But, as you age, your body produces less and less catalase, leaving a surplus of hydrogen peroxide.

**Reversing Gray Hair**

Now that we know why hair goes gray, the chances of developing a "treatment" for gray hair becomes much more likely. By increases the activity of enzymes that break down hydrogen peroxide while stimulating the producing of melanin (the pigment that colors hair), then gray hair may be a thing of the past.

**5. Preventing and Treating Age Spots**

Age spots are often the target of anti aging skin care products. There are some misunderstandings about age spots. First off, they are not caused by aging, but by exposure to the UV light of the sun. Sometimes people will call them "liver spots" though they have nothing to do with the liver. For me, there is something particularly gross about calling something on your hands a "liver spot." Maybe it's just a personal quirk, but I really don't like that term at all.

## Solar Lentigo – Age Spots by Another Name

The proper, and more useful, name for age spots is "solar lentigo." Basically this means a spot caused by the sun. Essentially, age spots are really big freckles and usually appear on the arms, face, hands, back and feet. People with fairer skin are more likely to get age spots. Age spots are not an appearance-issue only, because sometimes there is dryness, roughness and even thinning of the skin at the age spot (which could lead to increased bruising).

## Treatment for Age Spots

Effective age spot treatment is typically done by a dermatologist. There are several different approaches depending on the skin, location and number of age spots being treated. Some of the approaches use fade creams to lighten the area of the age spot. Other approaches attempt to freeze off the age spots using cryotherapy. There are also procedures to remove age spots using lasers and tretinoin (Retin-a and other products). All of these are done by prescription. You may find some over-the-counter creams that claim to fade age spots – they might work a little, but are much less potent than the prescription creams.

## Preventing Age Spots

Anti aging skin care for preventing age spots is pretty simple: Reduce your exposure to the sun. You can do this by avoiding exposure through wearing protective clothing and simply not being out in the sun too much. You can also prevent age spots by using sunscreens. Consider using a daily face and hand cream that has sunscreen in it. This would help prevent age spots on the most visible parts of your body.

## 6. Anti-Aging Skin Care Products, Problems and Solutions

Anti-aging skin care products flood the shelves with claims about reducing wrinkles and fading age spots. What is the truth behind these anti-aging skin care products? Why does skin age in the first place? What can you do to prevent skin aging?

### Sunscreen as an Anti-Aging Skin Care Product

Anti aging skin care products should all have one thing in common: sunscreen. Sun damage is behind almost all of the signs of aging skin such as wrinkles and age spots. To prevent damage to your skin from aging, be sure that sunscreen is your number one anti aging skin care product. Choose a sunscreen with an SPF rating of at least 15 (use a sunscreen with a higher rating if you plan to be in the sun for a longer period of time). Also, be sure that you use a broad-spectrum sunscreen that protects your skin from damage from UVA and UVB rays. Finally, be sure that your sunscreen is water resistant even if you are not planning on swimming -- your sweat alone undoes the protection of non-water resistance sunscreens. All the ointments, moisturizers and creams in the world can't compare to the anti aging effectiveness of ordinary sunscreen. Here are some other tips to keep looking young:

**Avoid the Sun:** Sunscreen is great, but if you can avoid long exposure to the sun that is even better. Don't spend a whole day at the beach in the beating sun. Limit your time out in the sun and your skin will age better.

**Wear Protective Clothing:** If you have to be in sun, do your best to keep the sun off your body. Wear long sleeved shirts and pants. A hat with a wide brim is great to protect your head and your face, neck and shoulders.

**Wear Sunglasses:** Your eyes can be damaged by UV light as well as your skin. Be sure to wear sunglasses that protect against 99% or more of UV rays.

**Avoid Artificial Tanning**: Sunlamps and tanning beds are just asking for trouble -- don't use them. They will damage your skin and speed your skins aging while increasing your risk for skin cancer. Artificial tanning lotions and make-up actually do provide some minimal protection from UV rays. But the effect is minimal and short-lasting. Your skin may look darker, but you have none of the protection of a real tan (and people often don't bother with sunscreen and tanning make-up together because it just ends up a creamy mess). Finally, avoid anything marketed as a tanning pill. These pills basically turn your skin orange and the long-term safety of high doses of tanning pills is unknown.

**Check Your Skin:** Almost of 50% of people who make it to age 65 will have skin cancer in their lifetime. You need to check your skin often for any signs of skin cancer as well as see a dermatologist regularly for a skin check. Learn how to do a skin self-check.

### 7. How Often Should Epsom Salts Be Used?

Epsom salts are salts that contain magnesium sulfate. When used in a bath, the magnesium sulfate is absorbed by the skin. This can cause the skin to soften and some of the substances that the skin absorbs day-to-day to be drawn out.

Occasional use of Epsom salts (especially on the feet) does not seem to be harmful. Many people swear by Epsom salts, though there doesn't seem to be many scientific references to its use. There are a few cautions of using Epsom salts, however, and they are mostly for people with dry skin.

The FDA doesn't seem very impressed with Epsom salts, even for foot care. They claim that Epsom salt foot baths show no benefit over soaking in a regular table salt bath in terms of softening the foot. They further caution that too much soaking in Epsom salt can cause excessive drying of the feet. People with diabetes and others with fragile skin are advised to soak in a foot bath with liquid dishwashing soap (the kind with skin softeners) instead.

The National Institute of Arthritis and Musculoskeletal and Skin Diseases (part of the NIH) does mention that an Epsom salt bath can help remove or soften any scaling that occurs with psoriasis.

In short, when using Epsom salts, be very careful about drying out the skin. Start with just a little (1/4 cup) in the bath, and gradually increase as needed. Monitor your skin closely for dryness. Try an Epsom salt bath once a week at first to see how your skin reacts. It may be that you need to avoid Epsom salt baths in the wintertime (when both the air and your skin tend to be drier), but can take them more frequently in the summer if you live in a humid location.

## 8. Top 10 Ways to Protect Your Beauty

**Avoid Sun Damage** - Tanning, sunbathing and overexposure do incredible harm to your skin. Not only does this increase your risk of skin cancer, but it also damages your skin. Freckling, wrinkles, and loss of elasticity all occur when your skin is overexposed.

**Don't Smoke** - Smoking will not only lower your life expectancy, it will make you look (and smell) bad. Smoking damages the skin in many ways:

Nicotine causes blood vessels to constrict, robbing skin of essential nutrients and oxygen. Recent research indicates that smoking activates an enzyme that breaks down collagen.

Wrinkles, fine lines around the mouth, stained teeth and fingers, and an overall "grayish" appearance to the skin all contribute to smokers often looking much older than their actual age.

**Drink Plenty of Water** - Proper hydration help the skin to stay firm and 'glowing'. To get a healthful look, be sure to drink plenty of fluids-- at least eight 8-ounce servings per day.

**Maintain Good Posture** - Slouchy people are not beautiful. Good posture and poise will help you to retain a 'look' of confidence and command. Improve your posture through exercises that focus on your core strength like yoga and Pilates.

**Take Sufficient Calcium** - Poor calcium intake leads to osteoporosis, a condition in which the bones of the body deteriorate. In severe cases, osteoporosis causes permanent hunching of the back, called kyphosis. Avoid this condition through assuring your calcium intake is sufficient by taking a supplement and including dietary sources of calcium.

**Smile and Laugh** - Happy people are beautiful. People who laugh and smile are attractive. Spread joy and happiness wherever you go and people will find you beautiful. Laughing and smiling can also help you to live longer. A positive attitude tells your body that 'everything is okay' and your body responds with the benefits of relaxation.

**Brush and Floss Your Teeth** - A good smile is important for beauty (see above), but you must work to maintain it. In addition, recent research has shown links between poor oral health and cardiovascular disease and diabetes. Flossing, regular dental check-ups and good dental habits will all help make your smile brighter. Avoid smoking and excessive coffee and tea to prevent staining.

**Appreciate Yourself** - People who like themselves are much more attractive than those who do not. Accept yourself for the wonderful person that you are. Your body language will improve and people will pick up on a confident 'vibe'. Much about beauty is perception and confidence. Start by convincing yourself, then others will follow suit.

**Eat Healthy Fats** - Healthy fats (from foods such as fish, nuts and avocados) containing essential fatty acids (EFAs) help your skin to look healthy and 'glowing'. A diet low in these healthy fats can result in problems such as eczema, dandruff, dull and brittle hair, and splitting nails. Be sure to eat these good foods to keep your skin and the rest of your body healthy.

**Stay Fit** - Of course having a fit, healthy body goes a long way to contributing to your looks. Excess weight, low muscle tone and lack of energy all contribute to a worsened appearance. Develop exercise habits that will last a lifetime to help you look better and live longer.

### 9. How is Inflammation Important to Aging?

Inflammation is caused by an immune reaction on the cellular level. It can be caused by infection or allergies, but also by many lifestyle factors including:

- smoking
- poor nutrition
- lack of sleep
- sun exposure

Inflammation has been linked to many things that we associate with aging, including wrinkles, arthritis, heart disease, Alzheimer's disease and cancer. Much inflammation can be reduced or prevented by changing our habits and environment or following an inflammation-reducing diet.

## I Have a Special Gift for My Readers

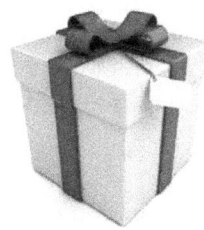

I appreciate my readers for without them I am just another author attempting to make a difference. If my book has made a favorable impression please leave me an honest review.    Thank you in advance for you participation.

My readers and I have in common a passion for the written word as well as the desire to learn and grow from books.

My special offer to you is a massive ebook library that I have compiled over the years. It contains hundreds of fiction and non-fiction ebooks in Adobe Acrobat PDF format as well as the Greek classics and old literary classics too.

In fact, this library is so massive to completely download the entire library will require over 5 GBs open on your desktop.

Use the link below and scan all of the ebooks in the library. You can select the ebooks you want individually or download the entire library.

The link below does not expire after a given time period so you are free to return for more books rather than clog your desktop. And feel free to give the link to your friends who enjoy reading too.

I thank you for reading my book and hope if you are pleased that you will leave me an honest review so that I can improve my work and or write books that appeal to your interests.

Okay, here is the link…

http://tinyurl.com/special-readers-promo

PS: If you wish to reach me personally for any reason you may simply write to mailto:support@epubwealth.com.

I answer all of my emails so rest assured I will respond.

**Meet the Author**

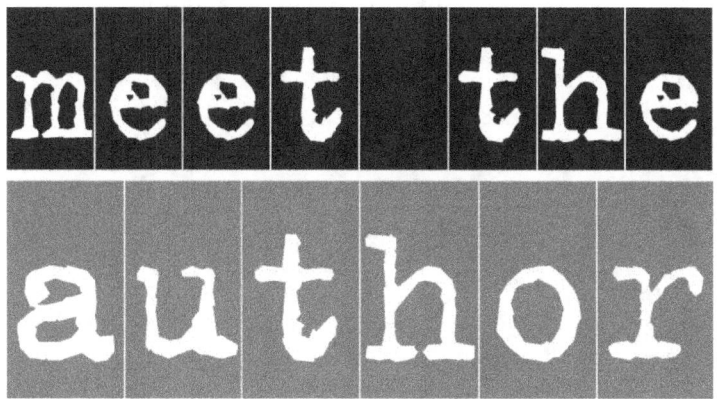

Dr. Noah Pranksky is a research behavioral scientist for Applied Mind Sciences. His research involves many aspects of the human mind including relationships, energy psychology, and various protocols and modalities relating to treatment and cure of various mental maladies.

He and his wife Marianne reside in Portland, Oregon.


**Visit some of his websites**
http://www.AddMeInNow.com
http://www.AppliedMindSciences.com
http://www.AppliedWebInfo.com
http://www.BookbuilderPLUS.com
http://www.BookJumping.com
http://www.EmailNations.com
http://www.EmbarrassingProblemsFix.com

http://www.ePubWealth.com
http://www.ForensicsNation.com
http://www.ForensicsNationStore.com
http://www.FreebiesNation.com
http://www.HealthFitnessWellnessNation.com
http://www.Neternatives.com
http://www.PrivacyNations.com
http://www.RetireWithoutMoney.org
http://www.SurvivalNations.com
http://www.TheBentonKitchen.com
http://www.Theolegions.org
http://www.VideoBookbuilder.com

www.ingramcontent.com/pod-product-compliance
Lightning Source LLC
Chambersburg PA
CBHW070441290526
45791CB00005B/2067